Internationale Not- und Katastrophenhilfe
Prof. Dr. Dr. Timo Ulrichs (Editor)

Tuberculosis out of control – strategies to fight multidrug-resistant tuberculosis

Akkon Schriftenreihe, Band 1
Akkon - Hochschule für Humanwissenschaften

akkon
hochschule für
humanwissenschaften

ISBN Angaben

978-3-945735-00-8

Imprint

Publisher

Prof. Dr. Dr. Timo Ulrichs
Akkon-Hochschule für Humanwissenschaften
Colditzstraße 34-36
12099 Berlin

Phone: +49 30 80 92 332-0
Fax: +49 30 80 92 332-30
info@akkon-hochschule.de
www.akkon-hochschule.de

Mit freundlicher Unterstützung der Janssen Cilag GmbH
und von Becton Dickinson Diagnostics

TABLE OF CONTENTS

Editorial
Timo Ulrichs
Akkon University for Human Sciences
Koch-Metchnikov-Forum **4**

Welcome remarks
Detlev Ganten
President World Health Summit **8**

Welcome remarks
Helmut Hahn
President Koch-Metchnikov-Forum **12**

The Berlin Declaration on Tuberculosis and its consequences for fighting multidrug-resistant tuberculosis in the WHO-European region
Timo Ulrichs **14**

The WHO European Region: Brief overview of the fight against Tuberculosis (TB)
Martin van den Boom **20**

A new model of collaboration and innovation to eliminate TB: The private company point of view
Adrian Thomas **30**

Advocacy in Tuberculosis
Stop-TB Forum **38**

Editorial

Timo Ulrichs

Editorial

„Tuberculosis out of control – strategies to fight multidrug-resistant tuberculosis" – A satellite symposium to the 5th World Health Summit in Berlin, October 21, 2013

In times of an acute global health emergency caused by a single infectious agent like the Ebola virus, public attention is drawn to infectious diseases and their control worldwide.

The ongoing catastrophe of the Ebola epidemic in Western Africa makes us rethink our abilities to fight infectious diseases with public health strategies as well as with research and development. However, despite imminentsituations of outbreaks like Ebola, Chikungunya or cholera, the chronic disasters and their impact on human development and welfare must not be forgotten: malaria, HIV/AIDS and tuberculosis are the three big killers of mankind and account for millions of deaths annually.

Enormous efforts have already been undertaken to get these infectious diseases under control, but still the fight against them requires an increasing resources worldwide. Especially tuberculosis control becomes more and more difficult as tuberculosis is aggravated by HIV coinfection in Subsaharan Africa, and the emergence of multidrug resistance mainly in the WHO-European Region causes still increasing numbers of patients. In recent years, the main problems of tuberculosis control in Africa and the WHO-European Region each were rising in the other region, respectively: South Africa reports more and more multidrug resistant cases, and in Eastern Europe an increasing HIV epidemic meets multidrug-resistant *Mycobacterium tuberculosis*, a very worrying situation.

The biggest challenge in fighting tuberculosis in the WHO-European Region remains the fast-growing rate of multidrug-resistant strains of *M. tuberculosis*. Multidrug-resistance, aggravated by an emerging HIV-epidemic in many of the successor states of the former Soviet Union, counteracts all efforts to efficiently control tuberculosis. In fact, we are more and more losing control, and tuberculosis has already become virtually untreatable in some areas of our WHO-European Region. Thus, the development of new drugs and novel vaccine candidates becomes more and more urgent. To address these challenges and to report the current state of the development of new drug and vaccine candidates, Koch-Mechnikov Forum and the Akkon University of Human Sciences organized a scientific symposium on the occasion of the World Health Summit in October 2013 with the aim of discussing these topics on a scientific, political and practical level and at the same time raising awareness of this imminent threat to global health.

The undersigned, who chaired the symposium, gave a brief introduction illustrating the current epidemiological and socio-economic situation. With state-of-the-art presentations, Steve Murray from TB Alliance (new drugs), Wanjiku Kamau from Aeras Global Vaccine Foundation (novel vaccine candidates) and Martin van den Boom from the WHO Regional Office (strategy paper on fighting multidrug-resistant tuberculosis) prepared the following panel discussion.

Together with the presenters, representatives from non-governmental organizations (Sebastian Dietrich from Médecins sans Frontières, and private companies, Adrian Thomas from Johnson & Johnson) contributed with their specific views on the issues of how to

- efficiently fight multidrug-resistant tuberculosis,
- develop new strategies,
- increase awareness,
- form alliances among all participating groups, namely governments of high and low burden countries, non-governmental and civil society organizations, media, academic and industrial partners.

The panel discussion was then opened to the audience (more than 50 participants followed the invitation), and enriched by various contributions. The scientific and political outcomes of the discussion were compiled and presented at the upcoming 8th Scientific Symposium of the Koch-Mechnikov Forum on the occasion of World Tuberculosis Day in Berlin, March 18 and 19, 2014, as well as submitted to both World Health Summit and WHO. It was also decided to ask the presenters to submit manuscripts of their contributions in order to publish a state-of-the-art review on tuberculosis control as the first issue of the Akkon-Schriftenreihe (periodical of Akkon University).

This publication is very timely as 2014 saw the launching of two urgently needed new anti-tuberculosis drugs, and with these two new weapons the fight against multidrug-resistant tuberculosis gets new support. However, if we want to keep the two drugs as efficient weapons, their implementation in high-burden countries and their subsequent application in combination drug regimens need to be rational. Public/global health strategies need to be applied, and consequent education and training programs for tuberculosis control personnel must ensure optimal knowledge transfer. Thus, Koch-Mechnikov Forum established a TB Training Center in Berlin and collaborates with partners in both microbiological diagnostics as well as the TB-drug developing pharmaceutical companies for optimal training courses.

This publication is also very timely as 2015`s G7 summit in Germany set the fight against global antibiotic resistances as top priority. Together with other organisations active in TB research and control, Akkon University and Koch-Metschnikov-Forum submitted a concept paper on how to fight the emergence of resistances, especially those of *M. tuberculosis.*

And Akkon University will consequently enlarge its portfolio of study programs, summer schools and expert fora with a special focus on global health and teach both chronic and acute infection control. Research and control of tuberculosis will form a special focus. This will ensure that students and young scientists will learn about the challenges of tuberculosis control and be able to efficiently fight the disease in the future.

Author

Prof. Dr. med. Dr. PH Timo Ulrichs

Akkon University for Human Sciences
Colditzstraße 34-36
12099 Berlin

Phone: +49 30 80 92 332-15
timo.ulrichs@akkon-hochschule.de

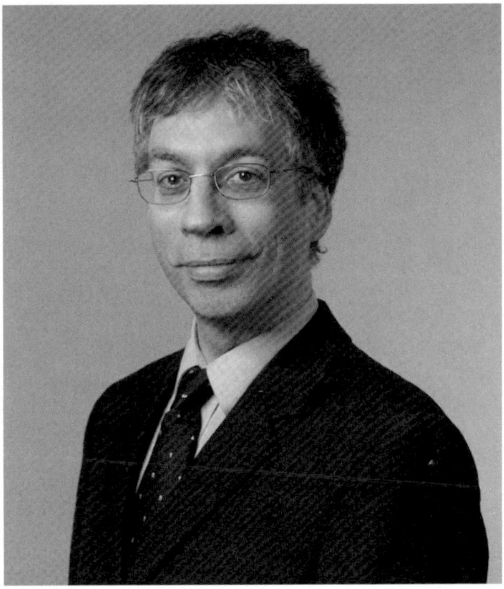

Welcome remarks

Detlev Ganten

Publication on the:

WHS Satellite Event 2013, hosted by the Koch-Mechnikov Forum

Welcome Message by:

Professor Detlev Ganten, Founding President of the World Health Summit

"Tuberculosis out of control – strategies to fight multidrug-resistant tuberculosis "

About 100 years ago, the famous German author Thomas Mann wrote his classic novel "Der Zauberberg" ("The Magic Mountain"), set in a sanatorium in the Swiss Alps where Tuberculosis was being treated. After centuries of causing millions of deaths worldwide, it was a time when this number one killer was effectively fought for the first time. Robert Koch had identified and described the bacillus causing Tuberculosis, *Mycobacterium tuberculosis*, on March 24, 1882, and sanatoriums were installed all over Europe. Tuberculosis was slowly fought back. Robert Koch received the "Nobel Prize in Physiology or Medicine" in 1905 for his discovery; Thomas Mann received the "Nobel Prize in Literature" in 1929. They were followed by Ilya Ilyich Mechnikov, the great Russian Scientist, who received the Nobel Prize in Medicine in 1908, sharing it with Paul Ehrlich from Germany.

Are we looking at a success story of Russian, German, and international cooperation, strongly supported by the Koch-Mechnikov Forum today? Yes and no. Attention and research turned to other diseases and existing TB treatments were not developed further, the disease changed and adjusted to existing medical means. Today, Multidrug-Resistant Tuberculosis is spreading and about one third of the world's population is still infected with Tuberculosis bacteria, as the World Health Organization (WHO) reports. Although only a small proportion of those infected will become sick with TB, 8.6 million people fell ill with it in 2012. It affects mainly the poorest of the poor, as people with weakened immune systems face the highest risk. They can hardly pay for the necessary treatment or the healthy lifestyle that keeps the immune system strong. Hence, the WHO estimates a need for two billion US dollars per year to fill the resource gap for implementing existing TB interventions. This money would need to be invested wisely and in a timely manner, as Multidrug-Resistant Tuberculosis is spreading rapidly. In the year 2012, more than 450,000 people developed this altered form of the disease that's becoming harder and harder to cure.

How can this challenge be met? The means developed a hundred years ago might not be working anymore, but the principles can still be applied: paying close attention to this widespread infectious disease and working together across sectors and across borders. This approach is not only the topic of the Koch-Mechnikov Forum symposium, but the core idea of the World Health Summit (WHS) as well. In 2009, the WHS was held for the first time and quickly became one of the world's foremost meetings for global health. It is effectively setting the global health agenda because it brings together international representatives of all involved areas: academia, politics, civil society, and the private sector. They work cooperatively on solutions in an atmosphere of academic freedom and mutual respect. Such a setting is required to attain results that draw from highly diversified expertise and simultaneously meet the real-life demands of all parties involved. It is the only angle from which Multidrug-Resistant Tuberculosis can be combatted successfully.

Multidrug-Resistant Tuberculosis is a perfect example for the complexity of fighting diseases in a globalized world and the necessity of joint reactions. It will not be addressed by market interests alone, because it still is a poverty associated disease. Non-Governmental Organizations (NGOs) are doing a great job to help, but they need strong political support. Again, the World Health Summit provides the perfect platform to meet this need. The health chapters of all national academies are organized in the Inter Academy Partnership for Health. Their mission is to report and advise their national governments on health related questions. This Inter Academy Partnership for Health is part of the M8 Alliance – the academic backbone of the World Health Summit. Thus, results can be communicated straight to governments worldwide to effectively influence their agendas. Successful examples of this procedure are the inclusion of climate change and its effects on health into political decision-making, and a call for action to strengthen research capacity building in low- and middle-income countries.

Since its inauguration in 2009, the World Health Summit has been closely working together with the Koch-Mechnikov Forum . Their satellite sessions are wonderful supplements to our program and a good tool to address tuberculosis in its various forms. I am very happy to see this cooperation not only continue, but vigorously grow, now also in collaboration with Akkon University. I cordially thank the Koch-Mechnikov Forum for their tireless work on this important topic and wish all participants from Russia, Germany and many other countries who are joining in, an interesting and successful meeting as well as a great experience at the World Health Summit 2014.

With best personal regards,

Detlev Ganten

Author

Prof. Dr. Detlev Ganten
President World Health Summit

WHS Foundation GmbH
c/o Charité-Universitätsmedizin Berlin
Charitéplatz 1
10117 Berlin

E-Mail: detlev.ganten@charite.de

Gemeinsam innovativ

Forschung und Entwicklung wird GROß geschrieben

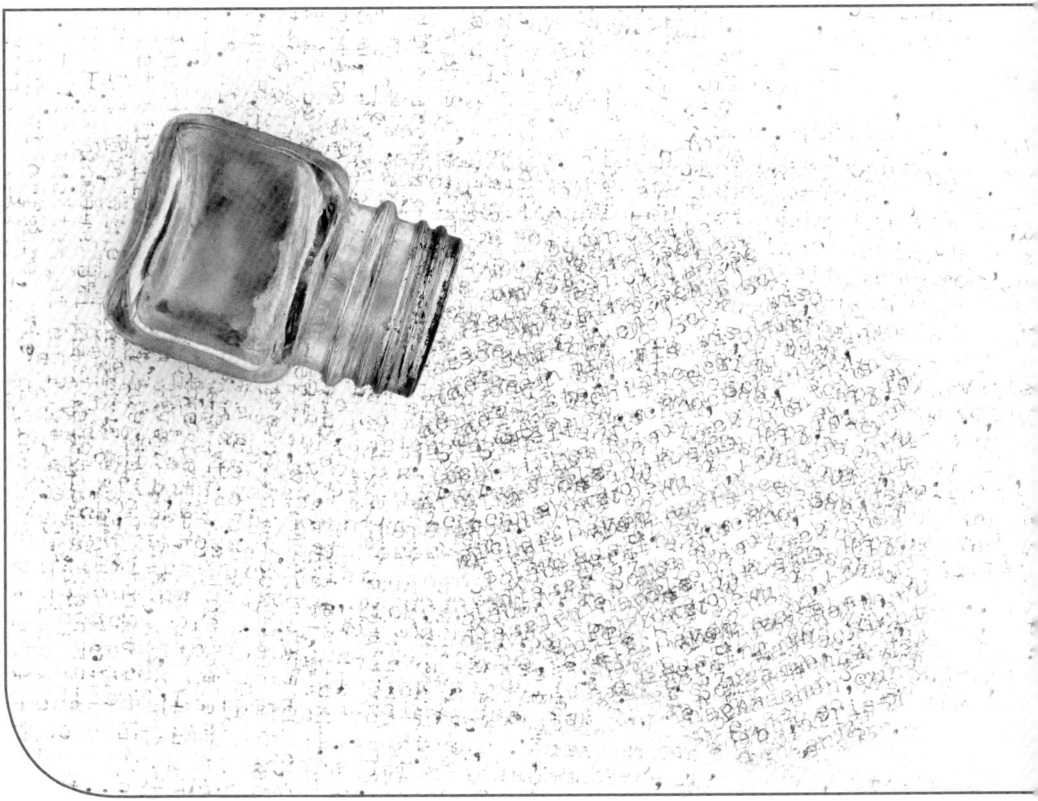

Die Akkon-Hochschule engagiert sich für Forschung und Entwicklung im Bevölkerungsschutz sowie in der Pflege. Unser Ziel ist es, mit unseren Partnern in anspruchsvollen Projekten zusammen zu arbeiten.

Die Studierenden werden aktiv in die Forschung und Entwicklung mit einbezogen.

Erfahren Sie mehr z.B. in :

- akkon aspekte Diskussionsreihe
- Akkon-Schriftenreihe

akkon
hochschule für humanwissenschaften

www.akkon-hochschule.de

Welcome remarks

Helmut Hahn

Dear colleagues, dear readers!

When asking those who are lucky enough to live in one of the industrialized and highly developed countries of Western Europe what they know about tuberculosis, one runs the risk of getting the surprised answer: „TB, a thing of the past." Clearly, this is grossly misleading and shows a profound misunderstanding of the problem. For TB is, despite the enormous efforts spent in terms of human and material resources, one of the most tenacious infectious diseases on earth still in existence and, in fact, is still one of the main killers worldwide.

The reasons for this are manifold; one of the main reasons has been, and still is, ignorance on the part of the medical community. The application of antituberculous drug regimens favouring the development of resistant strains of *M. tuberculosis* and the negligence in dealing with the basic rules of chemotherapy all play an important role in the process which has presented us with, e.g. the Beijing strain of *M. tuberculosis*.

What should be done? Clearly and laudably, some developed countries have picked up the barrel and contribute their share to combating the disease. Some countries even are specialized in fighting TB and are doing it very effectively. It is gratifying to see how international alliances have been formed and contribute, year after year, to the fight against TB. Research, education, and on-site experience are needed most, and this requires, in the first instance, money.

Germany, with its long tradition of research in infectious diseases, calls a lot of experience its own and, on the other hand, is saddled with relatively few patients. Germany, therefore, ideally is predestined to play a leading role in the battle against TB. Berlin in particular boasts a number of institutions of worldwide reputation in research on TB, such as the Robert Koch Institute of the Federal Government, the Max Planck Institute of Infection Biology, and others. It was for this reason that Koch-Mechnikov Forum was founded by a small number of medical microbiologists and infectious disease immunologists twelve years ago with the aim in mind of exporting research competence and practical expertise on TB from Berlin to countries which need such expertise most, i.e. South Africa and Eastern Europe.

We are proud to see that World Health Summit recognizes our activities by letting us present our work in the form of this Satellite Symposium. Koch-Mechnikov Forum , being an „initiative of the Petersburg Dialogue", not only mediates medical competence, but, in addition, is active in the political sphere spreading the message and opening the ears to the plea of the neediest.

We also have to overcome restrictions and obstacles which are unnecessary. For instance, it is not possible to transport, or mail, patients' materials for research and diagnosis across borders of certain countries. Koch-Mechnikov Forum has been fighting such archaic irrationality for years, but with little success so far.

Berlin is the city of Robert Koch who, in 1882, delivered his famous lecture about *M. tuberculosis* in the library of the Institute of Physiology of Berlin University. Also, the local spirit of the building in which he had done his work leading to the discovery and the means of identification of *M. tuberculosis*, are still in existence. May the spirit and the visions of Robert Koch be with us in our fight against TB as they were in the past! This will help in bringing about the success of this meeting and the subsequent publication of its contributions in this first issue of the publication series of the Akkon University for Human Sciences.

Helmut Hahn

Author

Prof. Dr. Helmut Hahn
Foreign Member of Russian Academy of Medical Sciences (RAMS)
President, Koch-Mechnikov Forum

Langenbeck-Virchow-Haus
Luisenstraße 59
10117 Berlin

E-Mail: hahn@kmforum.eu

The Berlin Declaration on Tuberculosis and its consequences for fighting multidrug-resistant tuberculosis in the WHO-European region

Timo Ulrichs

His famous presentation „Ueber Tuberculose" changed the view on tuberculosis as disease, identified *Mycobacterium tuberculosis* as etiologic agent and revolutionized the fight against the infectious disease in diagnosis, therapy and prevention. Robert Koch (1843 - 1910) gave this presentation in Berlin on March 24, 1882 (Gradmann, 2006). Exactly 100 years later, 1982, the International Union Against Tuberculosis and Lung Disease (IUATLD) proposed the 24th of March as „World Tuberculosis Day". Fourteen years later, in 1996, WHO confirmed this day as official day commemorating the disease and its victims as well as the endeavours to globally fight tuberculosis. In contrast to Robert Koch's expectations, the time between 1882 and our days could not be used to substantially reduce the global burden of tuberculosis disease (Migliori et al., 2007).

Diagnostics

Based on Koch's discoveries, microscopic diagnostics of acid-fast stained mycobacteria was developed for sputum diagnostics – it is still nowadays the gold standard in diagnosing the pathogen in potential TB patients. Koch's tuberculin served as a basis for a skin test, revealing contact of the immune system to mycobacteria – two blood tests using *M. tuberculosis*-specific antigens nowadays promise a more precise immunological diagnosis. However, skin and blood tests give no information on whether a contact to mycobacteria/*M. tuberculosis* resulted in latent or active TB disease or even complete clearance of the pathogen from the host. Microbiological diagnosis of tuberculosis is the main tool in successfully fighting the disease globally. In recent years, some progress was achieved in improving culture techniques of *M. tuberculosis*, and determining its presence in clinical specimens using molecular biological techniques, and combining both to identifying *M. tuberculosis* as well as getting information on drug sensitivity (McNerney et al., 2012).

Therapy

When it comes to treatment, progress is even more limited than in diagnostics. After discovery of the principle of chemotherapy, streptomycin was the first drug to be found effective against *M. tuberculosis*. Therapy failure because of monotherapy was followed by the launch of more anti-TB drugs in the 1950's and 60's. Since then, there was no more development of new „first line" drugs dedicated primarily to TB treatment. As multidrug resistance evolved, second line drugs were identified to act as last line of defence against the spread of MDR-TB. MDR- and XDR-TB are now spreading faster than ever, and soon, there will be virtually no effective anti-TB drugs available (Migliori et al., 2007; Nicolau et al., 2012; Raviglione et al., 2012). Some new candidates are in the pipeline. However, they are mainly based on already established functional mechanisms and thus are threatened to soon lose their efficacy.

However, 2014 saw the implementation of two new drugs, delamanid (Obsuka) and bedaquiline (Janssen). Their integration into treatment regimens gives some hope in the fight against MDR-/XDR-TB.

Prevention

Robert Koch's tuberculin, originally developed as vaccine candidate, turned out to be ineffective. *Mycobacterium bovis* BCG, a live vaccine, was introduced in the 1920's and is now the most widespread vaccine ever applied to mankind. Unfortunately, there is still an increase in new infections every year, and still about 1.6 million patients die from TB each year (Ulrichs, 2008). Prevention by a new vaccine candidate is very necessary, and some candidates are in the pipeline and will be clinically tested (actual overview in Ottenhoff, 2012). Vaccine trials, however, have the difficulty that the efficacy of the vaccine candidate will be proven only after decades, if protection of a vaccinated population can be shown. Evidence of protection by biomarkers would shorten this clinical study time tremendously, but up to now, there are no reliable biomarkers to be used in a TB vaccine setting (McNerney et al., 2012; Raviglione et al., 2012).

The current global TB situation is more than worrying.

In 1993, WHO declared TB a global health emergency, since incidence and prevalence numbers significantly increased over the past years. Since then, many attempts have been undertaken to globally fight the TB pandemic – without measurable success. Two world regions are mainly affected by TB: Sub-Saharan Africa and the WHO Euro region. Both regions struggle with complicating problems: in the African region, TB-HIV comorbidity is the predominant obstacle to a successful containment of the disease. *M. tuberculosis* and HIV help each other in furthering the clinical diseases.

In the WHO-European region, the emergence of multidrug resistance (MDR) significantly reduces the treatment success rate (Marx et al., 2009). In the past years, we observed the appearance of MDR-TB in Africa and a growing HIV/AIDS epidemic in the successor states of the former Soviet Union. Thus, treatment and epidemiological containment of TB are becoming more and more complicated (Raviglione et al., 2012; Lienhardt et al., 2012).

In order to address the increasing challenges in fighting TB in the WHO-Euro region, WHO and the German Federal Ministry of Health organized a Ministerial Forum on TB in Berlin in October 2007. Of 53 member states, 49 sent their health ministers, prime ministers or other high representatives to Berlin. At the end of the forum, the Berlin Declaration on Tuberculosis was adopted by the present ministers (Castell et al., 2010; WHO-Euro Office, 2012 [online]). The declaration names the main problems in containing TB in the WHO region, calls upon the member states to increase their involvement in TB control and lists self-commitments of high- and low-burden countries. At the end, it is stated that progress in fighting TB should be evaluated every two years (WHO-Euro Office, 2012 [online]).

In order to scientifically prepare the Ministerial Forum and at the same time to commemorate the 125th anniversary of Robert Koch's groundbreaking presentation „Ueber Tuberculose", the Koch-Mechnikov Forum (KMF) together with other TB organizations in Germany organized a scientific symposium on the occasion of World Tuberculosis Day in March 2007. The results of the symposium formed the basis of the discussion preparing the declaration. In turn, the Berlin Declaration on Tuberculosis is still nowadays the basis of all activities of the KMF in TB research and control in bilateral scientific projects with partners in Eastern Europe and Central Asia.

As the first scientific symposium on World Tuberculosis Day was successful, KMF decided to organize symposia every year in March on the occasion of World TB Day.

The following scientific symposia were organized by KMF on the occasion of World TB Day:

Year	Main focus
2007	125th anniversary of Robert Koch's presentation about tuberculosis; preparation of the Ministerial Forum in Berlin in Oct 2007
2008	Current research topics in diagnostics, therapy and prevention of tuberculosis
2009	Public health measures in tuberculosis control
2010	Exchange of expertise between the two world regions South Africa and Eastern Europe/Central Asia
2011	Fighting childhood tuberculosis; a symposium in the honour of Dr. Klaus Magdorf
2012	Five years after the Berlin Declaration: Evaluation of progress and obstacles; a festive symposium on the occasion of KMF's president Prof. Hahn's 75th birthday.
2013	Public private partnerships in diagnostics, therapy and prevention of tuberculosis
2014	HIV-TB comorbidity– current challenges and strategies
2015	Vaccine development and prevention strategies (together with TBVI)

Every single scientific symposium of KMF at World TB Day referred to the Berlin Declaration, even if the main focus of the symposium was different. All symposia were organized by KMF together with representatives of the WHO-Euro office. Some symposia were used to officially launch WHO reports on different subjects in TB control, such as the report on MDR TB.

KMF promoted the Berlin Declaration also at the World Health Summit (WHS [i]), which is organized by Charité University Medicine and its partners of the M8 Alliance every year in Berlin in October. 2009, at the first World Health Summit, a symposium was organized by KMF focussing on the evaluation of the progress made two years after the Ministerial Forum. The main topic of this symposium was HIV-TB comorbidity (Castell et al., 2010). Two years later, at the third WHS 2011, the evaluation of the progress made was presented with a political focus. The symposium on World TB Day 2012 focussed on the scientific evaluation and its epidemiological and Public Health outcomes (s.a., table with World TB Day symposia).

In every scientific symposium on the occasion of World TB Day, MDR-TB was an important topic. And as the relevance of MDR-TB for global health issues, for health policies and politics as well as for strategic health care planning is very high, it was decided to organize a satellite symposium to WHS 2013 with a special focus on multidrug resistance and its consequences for efficient TB control. Thus, KMF invited representatives from WHO as supranational organization (WHO-European Office, Copenhagen), from two research organizations in treatment (TB Alliance) and vaccine development (Aeras Global Vaccine Foundation), from private companies involved in TB research and development (Janssen, Neuss) and from NGOs dedicated to TB control (MSF, Berlin), in order to ensure an interdisciplinary multifocal panel discussion on public private partnerships and recent developments in fighting MDR-TB. The discussion at the satellite symposium organized at the DBB Forum Berlin, exactly six years after the Berlin Declaration on Tuberculosis highlighted the main challenges of and strategic solutions for MDR-TB with special focus on the WHO European Region.

i www.worldhealthsummit.org

As the challenges in fighting MDR-TB are representative for poverty-related infectious diseases in general and the strategies and plans to counteract the spread of the multiresistent pathogen are illustrative for interventions in global health programs and infectious disease control in general, it was decided to compile the main contents of the symposium of October 2013 into the first issue of the Schriftenreihe of Akkon University for Human Sciences.

Author
Prof. Dr. med. Dr. PH Timo Ulrichs

Akkon University for Human Sciences
Colditzstraße 34-36
12099 Berlin

Phone: +49 30 80 92 332-15
timo.ulrichs@akkon-hochschule.de

Literature

Castell S, Hauer B, Manissero D, Ulrichs T, Zaleskis R, Loddenkemper R. Berlin Declaration on Tuberculosis: High Level Follow-Up of High Priority Countries for TB Control in the WHO-EURO Region, Double Trouble or Double Success? Bringing Together Diseases and Programs' - a symposium report. Pneumologie. 2010 Jul; 64(7): 422-9.

Gradmann C. Robert Koch and the white death: from tuberculosis to tuberculin. Microbes Infect. 2006 Jan; 8(1): 294-301.

Lienhardt C, Glaziou P, Uplekar M, Lönnroth K, Getahun H, Raviglione M. Global tuberculosis control: lessons learnt and future prospects. Nat Rev Microbiol. 2012 May 14; 10(6): 407-16.

Marx FM, Skachkova EI, Son IM, Strelis AK, Urazova OI, Hahn H, Krämer A, Ulrichs T. Control of tuberculosis in Russia and other countries of the former Soviet Union. Pneumologie. 2009 May; 63(5): 253-60.

McNerney R, Maeurer M, Abubakar I, Marais B, McHugh TD, Ford N, Weyer K, Lawn S, Grobusch MP, Memish Z, Squire SB, Pantaleo G, Chakaya J, Casenghi M, Migliori GB, Mwaba P, Zijenah L, Hoelscher M, Cox H, Swaminathan S, Kim PS, Schito M, Harari A, Bates M, Schwank S, O'Grady J, Pletschette M, Ditui L, Atun R, Zumla A. Tuberculosis diagnostics and biomarkers: needs, challenges, recent advances, and opportunities. J Infect Dis. 2012 May 15; 205 Suppl 2: S147-58. Epub 2012 Apr 10.

Migliori GB, Loddenkemper R, Blasi F, Raviglione MC. 125 years after Robert Koch's discovery of the tubercle bacillus: the new XDR-TB threat. Is „science" enough to tackle the epidemic? Eur Respir J. 2007 Mar; 29(3): 423-7.

Nicolau I, Ling D, Tian L, Lienhardt C, Pai M. Research questions and priorities for tuberculosis: a survey of published systematic reviews and meta-analyses. PLoS One. 2012; 7(7): e42479.

Ottenhoff TH, Kaufmann SH. Vaccines against tuberculosis: where are we and where do we need to go? PLoS Pathog. 2012 May; 8(5): e1002607.

Raviglione M, Marais B, Floyd K, Lönnroth K, Getahun H, Migliori GB, Harries AD, Nunn P, Lienhardt C, Graham S, Chakaya J, Weyer K, Cole S, Kaufmann SH, Zumla A. Scaling up interventions to achieve global tuberculosis control: progress and new developments. Lancet. 2012 May 19; 379(9829): 1902-13. Erratum in: Lancet. 2012 Jun 16; 379(9833): 2242.

Ulrichs T. Immunology of tuberculosis and current status of vaccine development. Pneumologie. 2008 Mar; 62(3): 143-7.

Websites

WHO-Euro Office (2007): The Berlin Declaration on Tuberculosis.
[online]: www.euro.who.int/document/e90833.pdf [28.08.2014]

The WHO European Region: Brief overview of the fight against Tuberculosis (TB)

Martin van den Boom

Despite considerable progress made in the fight against TB in the WHO European Region, as illustrated by the attainment of target 8 of Millennium Development Goal (MDG) 6 (halting and beginning to reverse the incidence of TB by the end of 2015), it does not seem likely that the target of reducing TB prevalence by 50% compared with a baseline of 1990 is achievable. Another MDG-related Stop TB Partnership target, namely halving TB mortality compared to a 1990 baseline, will probably not be reached by the end of 2015 either. In 2013, there were an estimated 460 000 prevalent TB cases (range 350 000–590 000), equivalent to 51 (39–65) cases per 100 000 population. As for TB mortality in terms of absolute numbers, there were an estimated 38 000 TB deaths in the Region in 2013 (1).

When considering the treatment success rate of new smear-positive TB cases globally, it is striking that the success rate in the Region is lower than both the global average and the rates of the other five WHO regions (2). The highest rates of multidrug- and extensively drug-resistant (M/XDR) TB are found in the European Region. Since treatment for patients with M/XDR-TB is much more difficult and lengthy than for patients with drug-susceptible TB, favourable treatment outcomes are less likely. In response, and following WHO Regional Committee for Europe resolution EUR/RC61/R7 in September 2011, a Consolidated Action Plan to Prevent and Combat Multidrug- and Extensively Drug-Resistant Tuberculosis in the WHO European Region 2011–2015 was developed by the WHO Regional Office for Europe and partners (3). This "roadmap" harmonized national strategies to fight TB, building on seven areas of intervention with the aim of helping to reduce the spread of drug-resistant TB. In the next few years, the Region will continue to support Member States so as to ensure that efforts for a world free of TB will not dwindle. Currently, in line with the global post-2015 End TB Strategy (4) endorsed by the Sixty-seventh World Health Assembly in 2014 in resolution WHA67.1, the Regional Office is developing a follow-up regional TB action plan for 2016–2020, building on progress made so far and addressing remaining challenges.

TB epidemiology in the European Region

Despite noteworthy achievements in the Region as regards TB prevention and care, there is no room for complacency since TB accounts for over 40% of all mortality from communicable diseases and is the most common cause of death among people living with HIV/AIDS (5).

Overall, the picture as regards TB in the Region is mixed, making the prevention and care of TB challenging tasks. This heterogeneity is shown in the uneven distribution of the TB burden across the Region: in 2013, 84% of incident and 85% of prevalent TB cases, 90% of mortality caused by TB, 90% of TB/HIV co-infections and more than 99% of MDR-TB occurred in the Region's 18 high-priority countries (Armenia, Azerbaijan, Belarus, Bulgaria, Estonia, Georgia, Kazakhstan, Kyrgyzstan, Latvia, Lithuania, Republic of Moldova, Romania, Russian Federation, Tajikistan, Turkey, Turkmenistan, Ukraine and Uzbekistan) (Fig. 1).

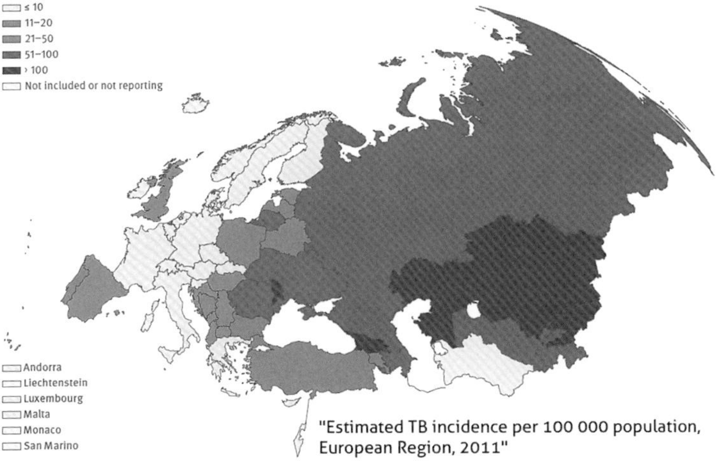

Figure 1: Estimated TB incidence per 100.000 population, WHO European Region 2013
Source: European Centre for Disease Prevention and Control/WHO Regional Office for Europe. (1)

By 2014, the overall treatment success rate for people with new and relapsed TB who started treatment in 2012 exceeded 75%. Fewer than 10 European Member States, however, reached or exceeded an 85% treatment success rate in this cohort (1). Some possible reasons for the comparatively low success rate are that:

- the TB/HIV co-infection rate has been rising in recent years;
- the European Region has the highest rate of MDR-TB of all the WHO regions;
- there have been challenges in maintaining an uninterrupted supply of high-quality TB drugs and challenges related to suboptimal TB management structures.

These conditions render TB more difficult to treat and favourable treatment outcomes less likely (2). Over half of the countries with the highest rates of M/XDR-TB in the world are in the eastern part of the European Region. This, combined with the fact that almost half of all previously treated TB patients develop M/XDR-TB, further explains the comparatively low treatment success rate (2). In addition, there has been a rising trend in MDR-TB among new cases and an alarming levelling out among previously treated cases in the Region (1). In 2013, limited laboratory capacity meant that only about 35 000 (46.6%) of an estimated 75 000 MDR-TB cases among notified TB cases were diagnosed. This, however, represented an improvement compared to 2012 (32 500, 42%) and to 2010, when only 36% of all estimated MDR-TB cases were diagnosed (1). Coverage of second-line TB treatment continued to improve in 2013. Reportedly more than 46 000 TB patients were enrolled in MDR-TB treatment. In some Member States, the number of patients enrolled exceeded the total notified because prevalent MDR-TB cases detected in previous years were still enrolled in treatment (Fig. 2).

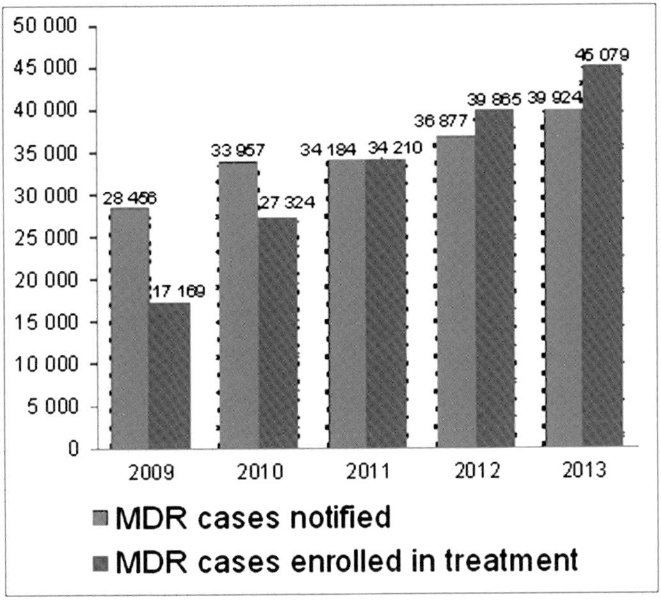

Figure 2. Trends in MDR-TB cases (i) notified and (ii) enrolled in treatment

The roadmap to prevent and combat drug-resistant TB

To combat TB and M/XDR-TB more efficiently, the Regional Office, in consultation with Member States, partners, civil society organizations and communities, developed the Consolidated Action Plan to Prevent and Combat Multidrug- and Extensively Drug-resistant Tuberculosis (M/XDR-TB) in the WHO European Region, 2011–2015 (3).

This plan was unanimously endorsed by the 53 European Member States in WHO Regional Committee for Europe resolution EUR/RC61/R7 in September 2011. The resolution urges Member States to harmonize, as appropriate, their national health strategies and/or national responses to TB and M/XDR-TB with the Consolidated Action Plan. One key goal of the plan is to contain the spread of drug-resistant TB by decreasing M/XDR-TB cases among previously treated cases by 20 percentage points, detecting 85% of M/XDR-TB patients and successfully treating at least 75% of MDR-TB cases.

Key progress and challenges in the Region

Further intensification of efforts is needed, based on the objectives in the Global Plan to Stop TB 2011–2015 (6), to reduce the burden of drug-resistant TB through several of the areas of intervention in the Consolidated Action Plan, such as preventing the development of M/XDR-TB, scaling up access to effective treatment and early diagnosis, improving surveillance and infection control, improving management capacity at national level and addressing vulnerable populations effectively.

In order to address and prevent further development of TB drug resistance, WHO assessed the reasons for defaulting from treatment in several settings. A TB/MDR-TB health system assessment tool has been developed and implemented in several Member States to document the key TB challenges to health systems and recommend mitigating measures. Even so, a key challenge remains in the inadequacy of treatment and patient support mechanisms in some Member States, including some in the European Union. Some Member States still require unnecessarily long hospitalization for TB patients which, without adequate airborne infection control, can lead to nosocomial transmission of drug-resistant forms of TB. Ambulatory services and other patient-centred and -friendly models of care, including home-based treatment, are being further expanded but are still not fully functioning in some Member States.

In an effort to improve countries' capacity, the Regional Office has assisted Member States to adapt and update their national MDR-TB and TB action plans. The Regional Green Light Committee for Europe, which has been providing technical support to European Member States in the clinical and programmatic management of drug-resistant TB, has also advised countries on effective responses to challenges related to TB drug resistance. To that end, the Regional Office and the European Respiratory Society have launched an electronic consilium in English and Russian enabling practitioners to consult on the clinical management of difficult to treat cases, particularly of X/- and MDR-TB patients.

With regard to the diagnosis and care of TB and M/XDR-TB, the Regional Office has established the European TB Laboratory Initiative and provided technical assistance to Member States to boost their diagnostic capacities and embark more systematically on improving the rapid molecular diagnosis of TB and MDR-TB. In addition, the Regional Office and other partners are continuing to provide technical assistance to improve collaborative TB/HIV activities, which will also contribute to increasing the detection of TB in people living with HIV/AIDS. Owing to reductions in domestic and international funding as a result of the global financial crisis, Member States have been facing considerable difficulties in expanding their diagnostic capacities and improving biosafety.

Low MDR-TB treatment success rates indicate that the tools and interventions currently in use should be employed more effectively, and would benefit from being complemented by new and more efficient measures. TB is one of the diseases that kill people living with HIV, and this deadly combination is increasing in the Region. The prevalence of HIV among TB cases increased from 3.4% in 2008 to 7.8% in 2013 (1). In 2013, less than 70% of TB patients had documented HIV test results and fewer than 55% of them were offered antiretroviral treatment (1).

Next steps and key foci in a nutshell

The Regional Office will continue to work with Member States and partners such as the European Centre for Disease Prevention and Control and the European Commission to increase awareness about the prevention and care of TB and MDR-TB.

Key focus areas are the scaling-up of good and best practices and patient-centred models of care, improvement in adherence to treatment, patient comfort and favourable treatment outcomes. Through efficient linkages with the Health 2020 policy framework (7), the social determinants of TB and M/XDR-TB will be more effectively addressed, leading to improvements in TB prevention and care in the Region. Greater attention needs to be paid to the strengthening of TB surveillance and bolder responses to reach out more effectively to risk groups and vulnerable populations, coupled with the careful introduction and rational use of new TB medicines under adequate and sufficient conditions of pharmacovigilance, so as to make further progress in TB prevention and care in the Region.
The further implementation of cross-border TB control and care and the development of interventions towards the elimination of TB in low TB incidence countries will be undertaken

to consolidate and expand progress and maintain achievements made to date. In addition, and strategically important, the Regional Office will assist Member States in implementing the global post-2015 End TB Strategy (4), which envisions a world free of TB, features ambitious goals and targets and builds on the following three key pillars:

i. integrated patient-centred care and prevention
ii. bold policies and supportive systems
iii. intensified research and innovation.

As stated above, the Regional Office is developing a regional TB Action Plan covering the period 2016–2020, in line with the global End TB Strategy and in collaboration and consultation with partners and Member States.

Author

Dr. Martin van den Boom

Technical Officer
Tuberculosis and
multidrug-resistant tuberculosis
Division of Communicable Diseases, Health Security and Environment

WHO Regional Office for Europe, Copenhagen, Denmark

References

1. Surveillance Report. Tuberculosis surveillance and monitoring in Europe 2015. Stockholm: European Centre for Disease Prevention and Control; and Copenhagen: WHO Regional Office for Europe; 2015 (http://ecdc.europa.eu/en/publications/Publications/tuberculosis-surveillance-monitoring-Europe-2015.pdf, accessed 29 May 2015).

2. Global Tuberculosis Report 2014. Geneva: World Health Organization; 2014 (http://apps.who.int/iris/bitstream/10665/137094/1/9789241564809_eng.pdf, accessed 29 May 2015).

3. Roadmap to prevent and combat drug-resistant tuberculosis. Copenhagen: WHO Regional Office for Europe; 2011 (http://www.euro.who.int/__data/assets/pdf_file/0014/152015/e95786.pdf, accessed 29 May 2015).

4. The End TB Strategy. Geneva: World Health Organization; 2015 (http://www.who.int/tb/post2015_TBstrategy.pdf, accessed 29 May 2015).

5. The European Health Report 2012. Charting the way to well-being. Copenhagen: WHO Regional Office for Europe; 2013 (http://www.euro.who.int/__data/assets/pdf_file/0004/197113/EHR2012-Eng.pdf, accessed 29 May 2015).

6. Stop TB Partnership. The Global Plan to Stop TB 2011–2015. Geneva: World Health Organization; 2010 (http://www.stoptb.org/assets/documents/global/plan/tb_globalplantostoptb2011-2015.pdf, accessed 29 May 2015).

7. Health 2020: a European policy framework supporting action across government and society for health and well-being. Copenhagen: WHO Regional Office for Europe; 2013 (http://www.euro.who.int/__data/assets/pdf_file/0006/199536/Health2020-Short.pdf?ua=1, accessed 29 May 2015).

A new model of collaboration and innovation to eliminate TB: The private company point of view

Adrian Thomas

Tuberculosis, especially the multidrug resistanttuberculosisisnotjustathreat for global health. It also has a negative effect on the long-term sustainable growth and economic development. To face these challenges it is necessary to do research and develop new drugs, treatment and diagnostic options. A close collaboration between the private, public and non-profit sector submit new innovative R&D concepts for drugs, treatment and diagnostic options. Equally important as the R&D are the timely diagnosis and appropriate use of drugs to prevent multidrug resistant tuberculosis. Here, the private sector can interfere by supporting national Governments to create sustainable and robust drug-resistant prevention strategies. At the end of the paper, the Janssen Company's contribution to the fight against TB is further explained.

Introduction

Innovation and collaboration are powerful tools to help people live healthier lives. This belief guides our efforts to tackle some of the world's most pressing health challenges and respond to unmet medical needs. Tuberculosis (TB) and especially multi-drug resistant tuberculosis (MDR-TB) is broadly recognized as an emerging threat to global public health (WHO, 2013 [online]). Significant progress has been made in the fight against the disease: the global TB mortality rate decreased 45 percent from 1990 to 2012 and, as a result, the United Nation's goal to halve the number of worldwide TB-related deaths by 2015 is within reach (WHO, 2013 [online]). But despite these significant gains, there is still much more work to be done. TB continues to cost countries and health systems dearly. Developing countries in particular continue to be disproportionally affected (TB Alliance, 2014 [online]). In 2012 alone, there were 8.6 million new cases of TB and 1.3 million TB-related deaths (WHO, 2013 [online]) – of these, 80 percent occurred in just 22 low and middle income countries (WHO, 2013 [online]).

Even more significant gaps remain in the diagnosis and treatment of MDR-TB. As TB bacteria become resistant to the most effective first-line TB medications, new treatments are needed that are often more costly, complicated, and toxic for patients (WHO, 2011 [online]). There were estimated to be close to half a million new cases of MDR-TB worldwide in 2012, and around 170,000 related deaths (WHO, 2013 [online]). But this burden is not shared equally. Today, 27 high-burden countries comprise around 85 percent of worldwide MDR-TB cases, with over half of these cases occurring in South Africa, China, India, and Russia (WHO, 2011[online]). Yet of the approximately 250,000 new MDR-TB cases per year

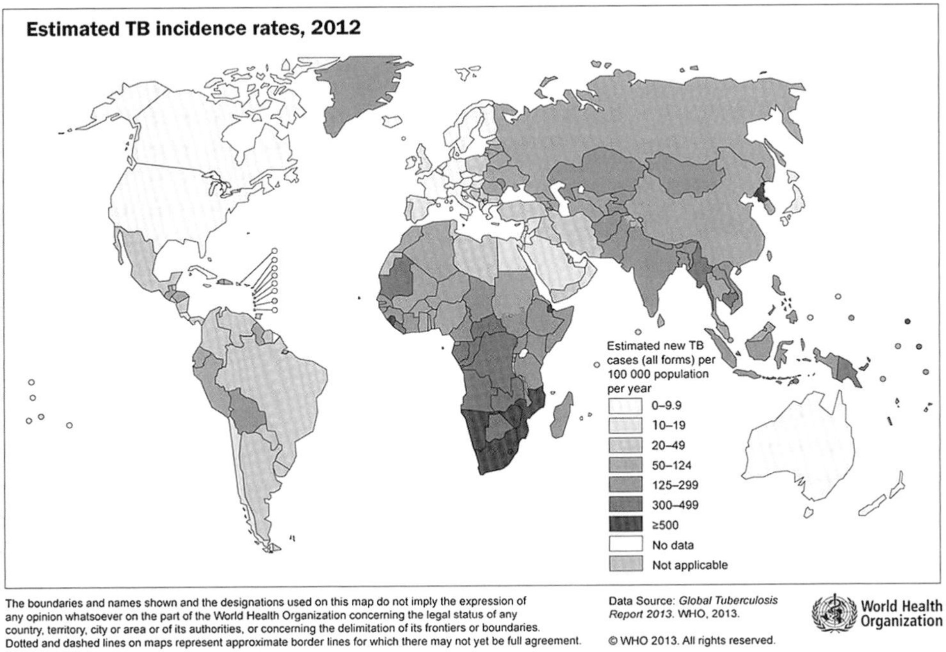

Figure 1 Estimated TB incidence rates

in these countries, only one in ten were reported to have started treatment (WHO, 2011 [online]).

Challenges and opportunities to cooperate

1. Investing in social and economic progress

As the world emerges from the economic downturn, governments are increasingly looking at better health as a means to ensure long-term sustainable growth and economic development. Investing to address TB and other infectious diseases must be an important element of this strategy recognizing that by some estimates, every $1 spent on TB diagnosis and treatment could generate as much as $30 in improved health outcomes and increased productivity (United Nations, 2013 [online]).

Studies have shown a close link between TB and poverty (TB Alliance, 2014 [online]). Underlying social determinants of health such as income inequality, social vulnerability, and inadequate housing expose people to an increased risk of contracting TB and developing drug resistance (WHO, 2009 [online]). There is considerable evidence to suggest that poor health, and TB in particular, prevents people from living long productive lives. Three-quarters of cases occur during the most productive ages of 15 to 54, contributing to losses of up to 30 percent of yearly household earnings (TB Alliance, 2014 [online]).

Moreover, TB places enormous strain on economies and health systems that could lead to reductions in Gross Domestic Product (GDP) by up to 7 percent (TB Alliance, 2014 [online]). In developing countries with already overburdened health systems, the situation is compounded by the fact that by 2015 as many as one million patients with MDR-TB will be in need of treatment (WHO/Stop TB, 2011 [online]).

The private sector has an opportunity to bring its financial and human resources, as well as its expertise, to the fight against some of the world's toughest and most intractable health issues. At Janssen, we have a legacy of working to address unmet medical needs including parasites, mycoses, diarrhea, and HIV/AIDS and the commitment to address neglected diseases drove us to develop the first medicine with a new mechanism of fighting MDR-TB bacteria in over forty years (Andries et. al., 2005). But drug discovery alone is not enough. As the threat from TB and MDR-TB continues to grow, greater collaboration between the private and public sectors, and new access and funding models for innovative R&D will be needed.

2. Driving innovation

Halting the rise of drug-resistant TB requires innovative new medicines and diagnostics that are effective, easy to use, and affordable. Yet the discovery and development of new treatments requires significant commitments of financial resources and the process can be lengthy. We need to find new ways to stimulate and incentivize R&D for diseases of the developing world such as MDR-TB. It is vital that these approaches diffuse the risks of drug development and delivery across the private, public and non-profit sectors. This means exploring a broader array of options for the de-risking of drug and diagnostic development, including advance market commitments, social-impact bond financing and prize models.

Advanced market commitments have shown promise in accelerating development timelines, providing stable (fixed) future demand and securing future pricing concessions. Social impact bonds involve a contract with government on "pay for success' terms - a commitment to fund interventions based on their public health impact. Such

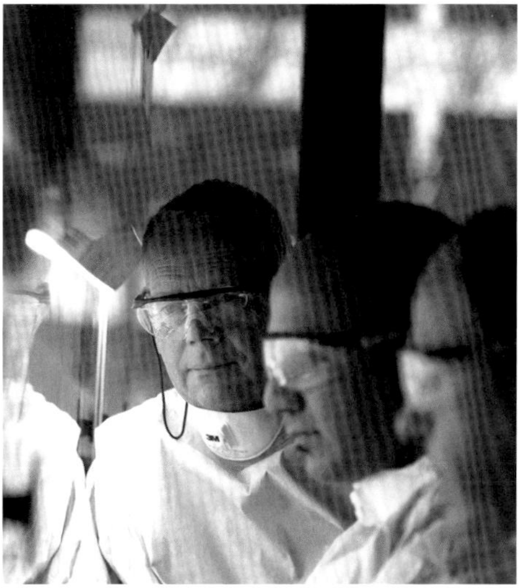

copyright: Janssen Cilag GmbH

public-private co-funding models have in the past proven successful in aligning fiscal incentives with health policy outcomes, while spreading risk. A 2011 report from the Center for American Progress notes they have the potential to improve results, overcome barriers to social innovation, and encourage investment in cost-saving preventative services (Liebman, 2011 [online]). For example, in March 2013, the City of Sacramento in the U.S. State of California announced that it was undertaking a project to design and launch the country's first "health impact bond" for interventions to improve patient care for children with asthma – which costs the city $35 million a year (Roosevelt Institute, 2013 [online]).

Collaboration is also critical if we are to make a meaningful difference to the lives of people with TB. Janssen is partnering with various entities, including: the TB Alliance on drug development; the Critical Path to TB Drug Regimens (CPTR) to accelerate new drug regimens; Stop TB Partnership to build awareness of the disease; and the Global Drug Facility to facilitate access to treatment, among others (Janssen Therapeutics, 2009 [online]).

3. Promoting timely diagnosis and appropriate use

Although innovative R&D is an essential component of the fight against TB, the development of new treatment and diagnostic options is only one piece of the puzzle. We also must ensure these medicines are used correctly to prevent the growing number of cases of MDR-TB. In 2012, less than a quarter of the people estimated to have MDR-TB were identified both globally and within most high-burden countries (WHO, 2013 [online]). Global roll-out of GeneXpert® technology for detection of MDR-TB as part of the World Health Organization (WHO) TBXpert Project has significantly improved the timely diagnosis of TB and MDR-TB. However, even as rates of diagnosis have ramped up in recent years, treatment is lagging behind. Only about three percent of MDR-TB patients are receiving treatment in line with WHO standards – and a large part of this missed opportunity can be attributed to health system weaknesses – especially in developing countries – and ineffective national TB treatment policies and programs (WHO, 2009 [online]).

Efforts to scale up national and community-based TB-related infrastructure should be redoubled. Ineffective drugs hamper treatment outcomes and exacerbate the proliferation of drug-resistant bacteria. Encouraging appropriate and responsible use of new drugs can help mitigate the acquisition of drug resistance and remains the most effective strategy for prevention and control of MDR-TB, which often results from treatment mismanagement or transmission from other patients (WHO, 2011 [online]).

The costs of inaction are enormous. Treating a single case of MDR-TB may cost as much as half a million dollars – ten times more than treating a drug-sensitive TB patient. Governments that fail to invest in their health care system and TB treatment programs now will undoubtedly end up paying more in future. Janssen is engaging developing and developed country governments – with both a high and low burden of TB – to address the challenges of ensuring appropriate use of first- and second-line treatments. These consultations highlight the vital need for national drug-resistance prevention strategies that can turn the tide of the MDR-TB epidemic. In this and many other areas, the private sector has a role to play in working with government to ensure these strategies are both robust and sustainable

Building a new approach to global health

To build on our work in addressing the world's greatest unmet public health needs, we recently formed Janssen Global Public Health (Janssen GPH), a new group devoted to utilizing the company's science and access models to drive better health outcomes, improve patients' quality of life, and sustainably advance health for people worldwide. Janssen GPH will initially focus on clinical and product development for health needs affecting emerging markets and resource limited settings.

At the forefront of this effort is our new treatment for MDR-TB, approved in the U.S. and Russia as part of combination treatment for MDR-TB, with a positive Committee for Medicinal Products for Human Use (CHMP) opinion released in December 2013. We are working to ensure patients have access to this medicine by creating responsible access and distribution plans. We have prioritized registration efforts in high disease burden countries, established a transparent equity-based pricing approach, and are working to forge novel forms of collaboration with public and private organizations. We recently announced a partnership with the Stop TB Partnership's Global Drug Facility (GDF) to support responsible introduction and appropriate use of our MDR-TB treatment in high-burden countries, including South Africa and India. And we're initiating a multi-country registry of high burden countries which, upon successful registration, will be eligible to participate in operational research in coordination with the WHO policy implementation package. It is hoped that this research will generate high quality TB treatment outcomes to inform policy guidance in the future.

Janssen GPH is also supporting research aimed at developing simpler treatment regimens and a robust pediatric study of child-friendly formulations. These and other efforts demonstrate our commitment and aspiration to deliver sustainable, long-term solutions that foster a greater sense of urgency in containing this deadly disease.

The way forward

We cannot stand by and allow future generations to bear the burden of this disease. Doing so will cost lives and even more money. As the 2015 deadline for the World Health Assembly universal TB treatment and access target is fast approaching, it is time to scale up the global response to TB and accelerate our efforts to meet the needs of patients. We believe that new models of collaboration and innovation, anchored by an innovative approach to R&D and a concerted effort to provide responsible access to treatment for those most in need, are urgently needed. Patients are waiting - it is our responsibility to deliver.

Author

Adrian Thomas

Adrian Thomas, M.D. Vice President Global Market Access, Commercial Strategy Operations and Global Public Health

Janssen Pharmaceutica NV 2014, Turnhoutseweg 30, B-2340 Beerse - Belgien

E-Mail: athoma15@its.jnj.com

Literature

Websites

Janssen Therapeutics (2009): Unique collaboration between TB Alliance and Tibotec to accelerate Tuberculosis drug development. In News, [online]: http://www.jnj.com/news/all/20090617_110000 [26.07.2014]

Liebman, Jeffrey B. (2011): Social Impact Bonds: A promising new financing model to accelerate social innovation and improve government performance. Center for American Progress, [online]: http://cdn.americanprogress.org/wp-content/uploads/issues/2011/02/pdf/social_impact_bonds.pdf [26.07.2014]

Roosevelt Institute (2013): Can Social Impact Bonds Unlock Private Money for Public Goods? Innovation in Pay-for-Success and Social Finance. Policy Note, [online]: http://rooseveltinstitute.org/sites/all/files/Keohane_Social_Impact_Bonds.pdf [26.07.2014]

TB Alliance (2014): Economic impact of TB, [online]: http://www.tballiance.org/why/economic-impact.php [26.07.2014]

United Nations (2013): A new global partnership: Eradicate poverty and transform economies through sustainable development (p. 39). [online]: http://www.un.org/sg/management/pdf/HLP_P2015_Report.pdf [26.07.2014]

WHO (2009): The Beijing „Call for Action" on Tuberculosis control and patient care: Together addressing the global M/XDR-TB Epidemic. Beijing, China: A Ministerial Meeting of High M/XDR-TB Burden Countries. [online]: http://www.who.int/tb_beijingmeeting/media/en_call_for_action.pdf?ua=1 [26.07.2014]

WHO (2011): MDR-TB and XDR-TB 2011 progress report. [online]: http://www.who.int/tb/challenges/mdr/factsheet_mdr_progress_march2011.pdf [26.07.2014]

WHO (2013): Executive summary. In Global Tuberculosis report 2013 (p. ix). [online]: http://apps.who.int/iris/bitstream/1665/91355/1/9789241564656_eng.pdf [26.07.2014]

WHO/Stop TB. (2011): The global plan to stop TB 2011-2015. Geneva: World Health Organization (p. 13). [online]: http://www.stoptb.org/assets/documents/global/plan/TB_GlobalPlanToStopTB2011-2015.pdf [26.07.2014]

Newspapers

Andries, K., Verhasselt, P., Guillemont, J., Gohlmann, H., Neefs, J., Winkler, H., . . . Jarlier, V. (2005): A diarylquinoline drug active on the ATP synthase of Mycobacterium tuberculosis. Science, 307(5707), 223-227.

Advocacy in Tuberculosis

Stop-TB Forum

Although Tuberculosis (TB) is one of the most widespread infectious diseases in the world it remains under-researched and in political discussions a neglected subject. Affecting mostly people of low socio-economic backgrounds, TB is a poverty associated disease and fraught with stigma. Non-governmental Organizations (NGOs)[i] can help to give TB-patients and their needs a voice by means of advocacy work. The following text will give a brief introduction to TB-advocacy, describing from a normative perspective the possibilities as well as the risks of NGOs advocating in TB. Special focus will be given to the role of advocacy-actors from non-high burden countries. As one example the work of the German advocacy-network "Stop-TB Forum" will be introduced.

i In the following NGOs are understood as all non-state actors who are not profit-oriented.

1. Advocacy - possibilities and risks

In globalized politics advocacy-NGOs can fill a gap between state and economy playing the role of a "watchdog". But there are also critical aspects connected with the involvement of advocacy-NGOs in politics that especially resource-rich NGOs of high-income countries in the northern hemisphere should be aware of.

There are a lot of definitions for the term "advocacy". Rooted originally in law, most dictionaries define advocacy as the process of 'speaking on behalf of someone'. Undertaken by NGOs, advocacy does not only speak on behalf of someone but also seeks change. A good definition for advocacy work of NGOs would be 'the process of using information strategically to change policies that affect the lives of disadvantaged people'. [ii]

ii Water Aid (2001): Advocacy. What's it all about? P.9, online: http://www.wsp.org/Hygiene-Sanitation-Water-Toolkit/Resources/Readings/WaterAidAdvocacy-all-sections.pdf [09.04.2014].

Advocacy-NGOs point to misconducts of state and economy and seek in some kind of way alteration. This alteration can be moderate or more or less radical and may be in policies and laws themselves, in the implementation of these policies, or even in people's awareness of the policies and their own rights.

The range of activities of advocacy-NGOs is extensive. Broadly, advocacy-NGOs can

1. inform the public about problematic aspects in politics and sensitize it;
2. inform political actors and lobby for change;
3. conduct relevant research as experts of specific topics and serve as a critical observer;
4. empower marginalized communities by transferring resources and giving them and their needs a stage.

An important aspect of advocacy work is the involvement of those communities advocacy-NGOs claim to speak for. This aspect in particular has been criticized especially when it comes to resource-rich NGOs from higher-income countries: Do NGOs really act in the best interests of those they advocate for? Competing for public attention and financial resources, agendas of NGOs are to a certain degree an end in itself so NGOs more often than not have conflicts of interests. And also without the aspect of self-preservation, the question of who has the power of definition still remains. Because even if NGOs have the best intentions, it does not necessarily mean that their views are in accord with those of people affected by the problem. Advocacy-NGOs should always be aware of their privileged position and their power of definition.

Another point of critique often raised is the democratic deficit of NGOs. Unlike political leaders they are not elected and thus not legitimized. Therefore NGOs should always try to be as transparent as possible so that everyone can reconstruct the basis of their argumentation and assess the potential influences over the NGOs. It is also important that if transferring any kind of resources, NGOs should not weaken the public sector as the latter one has to be included for sustainable and democratic solutions. [iii]

iii For a more comprehensive overview about problematic aspects of NGOs getting involved in politics see for example: Brunnengräber, Achim/Klein, Ansgar/Walk, Heike (Ed.) (2005): NGOs im Prozess der Globalisierung. Mächtige Zwerge – Umstrittene Riesen. Wiesbaden: VS Verlag.

In summary, in order to achieve accountability advocacy-NGOs should strive to provide:

a) transparency of the evidence base they use, of funding and funders for specific campaigns and activities, and of their overall goal and strategy;
b) inclusion to the affected and marginalized people they advocate for;
c) a critical evaluation and reflection of their work and its impact. [iv]

2. Tuberculosis – what is the problem?

As a poverty disease TB is among the neglected diseases. Although it is one of the widest spread diseases in the world and kills over one million people every year there has been little research in TB over the last decades. There is still no effective vaccination against it and with the spread of resistant forms of TB-bacteria there is a lack of sufficiently effective and well tolerated TB-medicine. Broadly, three areas of problems can be identified:

iv Hammer, Michael (et.al.) (2010): Addressing accountability in NGO advocacy, One World Trust, online: http://www.oneworldtrust.org/csoproject/images/documents/Self_regulation_of_advocacy_among_NGOs_OWT_125_March_2010_-_final.pdf [04.04.2014].

1. Lack of control and treatment of TB

The World Health Organization (WHO) estimates that 3 million people who had TB in 2013 were "missed" by health systems.[v] They were either not diagnosed or did not receive an accurate treatment, or sometimes none at all. This, however, does not only violate the human right for health of millions of people. As TB is an airborne disease the large number of "missed" TB-cases is also a great danger for the global control of TB.

Another problem for the control of TB is the high comorbidity-rate of TB and HIV/TB. 13% of all new TB-cases last year were also infected with HIV/Aids.[vi] Health facilities are often not well equipped for patients having both infections. Diagnosing and treating patients with TB and HIV is much more complicated as there is a lack of effective and coordinated methods.

2. Lack of development and research in TB

Due in part to incomplete and inconsistent treatment resistant forms of TB-bacteria have developed. The multidrug-resistant TB (MDR-TB) not only causes a serious drain on health systems, costing 10 to 15 times as much to treat as regular TB, MDR-TB also means more suffering for the patients.

v WHO (2014): World Tuberculosis Report 2014, online: http://bit.ly/1IH7JLF [18.05..2015].
vi Ibid.

Patients with this form of the disease must complete a two year course of powerful drugs that cause constant nausea and can leave them blind or deaf. Also the chance of recovery is still only 60%. [vii]

In the last decades there has been some progress in TB-research. For the first time in 40 years there are two new TB-drugs on the market. Although this is good news, it is not enough. As the treatment of TB includes at least four drugs there is an urgent need of new regimen. It is not yet known how and in which combination the new drugs shall be applied. If the new drugs are used inadequately, there is the possibility that new drug-resistance strains will develop.

Furthermore, there is a lack of effective and easy methods for diagnosing TB and there is still no effective vaccine against the disease which is urgently needed for a sustainable control of TB.

3. **Lack of effective measures against the social causes of TB**

As previously mentioned, TB especially affects communities with low socio-economic backgrounds. People living or working in environments that are unhygienic or poorly ventilated as well as people who are malnourished or have a weakened immune system are at much greater risk of being infected and developing active TB. The highest rates of TB are found in prisons and in mines.[viii] Sustainable control of TB has to take into account these social causes of the disease.

3. Advocacy in TB

Considering that TB is a preventable and curable disease the international TB-community demands „zero TB deaths, zero new TB infections, and zero TB suffering and stigma".[ix] Taking into account the above mentioned possibilities and risks of advocacy, what can advocacy-NGOs do to support this vision? Who should be addressed and with whom should NGOs cooperate in order to effectively fight TB? [x]

1. **Inform the public about the problematic aspects of TB**

By informing the public about the aforementioned problems concerning TB, advocacy can raise awareness for the global health threat the disease poses. An increased awareness of TB in high-burden countries as well as in countries where TB is thought to

vii WHO (2013): World Tuberculosis Report 2013, online: http://ow.ly/r2xbz [20.11.2013].

viii See for example: Stassen, lma (2012): TB- Miners hardest hit, in: Third World Resurgence No. 261, May 2012, pp 6-7, online: http://www.twnside.org.sg/title2/resurgence/2012/261/health1.htm [02.04.2014] and WHO (2005): Addressing poverty in TB control, online: http://www.who.int/tb/publications/tb_2005_352_tb_poverty.pdf [04.04.2014].

ix The Zero Declaration (2012), online: http://www.treatmentactiongroup.org/tb/advocacy/zero-declaration [02.04.2014].

x The following proposals of actions in TB-advocacy are in no way intended to represent a comprehensive list.

be "defeated" is not only an important factor when considering the spread of MDR-TB worldwide. Through awareness raising advocacy can also increase political pressure and change the stigmatizing image of the disease.

2. Inform political actors and lobby for change

In the pursuit of change advocacy has to address political decision makers. Regarding TB, advocacy-NGOs can point to TB-declarations within the framework of the WHO in which states have committed themselves to engage in the fight against TB.[xi] NGOs should inform political decision makers about the threat the disease poses and appeal to their governments to honor their commitments.

TB-advocacy should point out to decision makers that an increased engagement in the fight against TB cannot only mean increasing the contribution to the Global Fund to Fight Aids, Tuberculosis and Malaria (GFATM). Although the GAFTM is not sufficiently funded and does need more financial commitment, the fight against TB needs a more comprehensive answer. Looking at the above identified problems, such a respond should include a strengthening of health systems worldwide, more research and development in TB and measurements against the social causes of TB.

Advocacy-NGOs from high-income countries should demand a better inclusion of health and TB in the development cooperation from their governments. National TB programs should be supported and included in programs for health system strengthening. Additionally, advocacy in TB, as well as in any other poverty disease, should not only focus on aspects of health systems alone. As TB is highly connected with social conditions, a sustainable fight against the disease must include broader measures aiming at improvements of living and working conditions. NGOs should examine these structural connections and present solutions.

Furthermore NGOs should point out the problematic situation of many TB-patients in middle-income countries. The GFATM is planning to exit these countries because of their overall income. Many of these countries, like Russia, India and China, have a very high TB-burden. The overall income of these countries does not reflect that most of the poorest people in the world live in middle-income countries.[xii] Many of the people with TB in middle-income countries do not get the help they need due to poorly functioning health systems or stigmatization.

xi See for example. „The Berlin Declaration on Tuberculosis", WHO Europe, 2007, online http://www.euro.who.int/__data/assets/pdf_file/0008/68183/E90833.pdf [20.03.2014].

xii Sumner, Andy (2011): The New Bottom Billion: What If Most of the World's Poor Live in Middle-Income Countries? CGD Brief, online: http://www.cgdev.org/sites/default/files/1424922_file_Sumner_brief_MIC_poor_FINAL.pdf [02.04.2014].

As mentioned above, there is a lack of effective and well-tolerated TB-medicine. Advocacy in TB has to point out the suffering of MDR-TB-patients and demand more financial investments in TB-research and development. If sustainable solutions are sought, advocacy in TB should also point out the structural problem of neglected diseases and present alternatives. The lack of research in TB results from the fact that investments in research and development of pharmaceutical companies are refunded through the price of the developed products. This leads to the situation that pharmaceutical companies only provide research on diseases that affect people who have the money to pay for the drugs. There already exist a lot of proposals how the problem of lack of research in poverty-related diseases can be overcome, which advocacy-NGOs can present to political decision makers. [xiii]

3. Conduct relevant research and serve as a critical observer

As experts advocacy-NGOs can disclose correlations and develop alternatives. TB-advocacy might for example reveal the actual spending for TB worldwide, investigate the effects of patents for special TB-drugs or examine the social causes of TB. Such research is needed in order to underpin the critique raised by NGOs and to present alternatives to political decision makers.

TB-advocacy can also play an important role as an observer in research. Monitoring research trials, NGOs can make sure that affected people are included in the research process so that products are designed in consideration of those in need. For example, the Global TB Community Advisory Board[xiv] identified as an important concern for patients that the two newest TB-drugs cause complications if taken together. The advisory board called on the drugs' sponsors to cooperate in order to establish if the drugs are safe to use together. As a result, a study is now conducted to test the interaction of the two new TB-drugs. [xv]

TB-advocacy can also make sure that drugs are affordable and accessible for everyone in need. For punctual solutions they can demand drug donations or lower prices for urgently needed drugs from pharmaceutical companies.

xiii Some of them have already been partially implemented like the so called Product Development Partnerships (PDPs). PDPs combine different kinds of actors and aim at promoting research and development for neglected diseases. In recent years there has been a lot of progress in the TB drug pipeline due to PDPs. For an overview see: BUKO Pharma-Kampagne et al (2011): Forschung für vernachlässigte Krankheiten, Pharma-Brief spezial, online: http://www.bukopharma.de/uploads/file/Pharma-Brief/2011_02_spezial_Forschung.pdf [04.04.2014].

xiv The Global TB Community Advisory Board is an independent group of highly research-literate activists from global networks for HIV and tuberculosis.

xv See: DeLuca, Andrea (2014): The evolving role of advocacy in tuberculosis, in: The Lancet Respiratory Medicine, Volume 2, Issue 4, p. 258 – 259.

4. **Empower marginalized communities**

As mentioned above, advocacy-NGOs, especially those from non-high-burden-countries, should always make sure that their critiques and demands are fed back to the needs of affected communities. They should closely work together with affected people and coordinate their campaigns with international TB networks in which affected people are integrated. In contrast to other diseases like HIV/Aids only a few survivors of TB have served as public voices for it. This is partly due to the persistent stigma of TB worldwide, and the lack of funding to support community involvement in TB research and programs.[xvi] TB-advocacy has to make sure that affected communities are empowered to engage effectively in the fight against the disease. This can be achieved through training courses as well as financial support for example.

Considering that TB is highly connected with HIV/Aids, TB-advocates also ought to work together with advocates in HIV/Aids and health in general, so that measures against TB are integrated in a broader health context.

In order to increase political pressure, advocacy-NGOs should seek broad alliances. But NGOs should always consider the consequences a specific cooperation might bring about. The actual cause should not be left behind because of pragmatic alliances. For example, although political leaders will always tell TB-advocates that for a pragmatic solution the pharmaceutical industry should be involved, advocacy-NGOs should be aware that cooperation with pharmaceutical companies might jeopardize TB-advocacy-work for more sustainable solutions.

xvi Ibid.

The Stop-TB Forum – TB-advocacy in Germany

In 2009 the Stop-TB Forum was founded as a TB-advocacy network by German medical, humanitarian and development NGOs whose aim is to fight TB worldwide.

The network was founded against the background that in Germany TB is not recognized as a global health problem. The German public as well as most of German politicians consider TB as a controllable and, at least in Germany, "defeated" disease. The Stop-TB Forum primarily aims at raising awareness for the danger the infection poses as well as the needs of affected people. Furthermore it seeks an increased engagement of the German government in the global fight against TB. In consideration of the threat of TB as well as Germany's resources, the Stop-TB Forum considers Germany's role in the global fight against TB as insufficient. As the third biggest economy in the world and with its great capacity for research the Stop-TB Forum seeks an increased engagement of Germany and demands from the German government:

- a greater inclusion of TB in the German development cooperation,
- measurements targeting the social causes of TB
- more investment in development and research for TB
- help to secure universal access to TB-care for everyone in need.

The Stop-TB Forum

a) coordinates the work of the member organizations and engages in international networks

As the member organizations of the Stop-TB Forum work in different fields in the fight against TB they have different expertise to offer. The network connects actors who treat TB-patients in Germany as well as in high burden countries, NGOs who work closely together with patient organizations in high burden countries and actors with extensive backgrounds in TB research and critical observation of the pharmaceutical industry. Bringing together these different kinds of actors not only

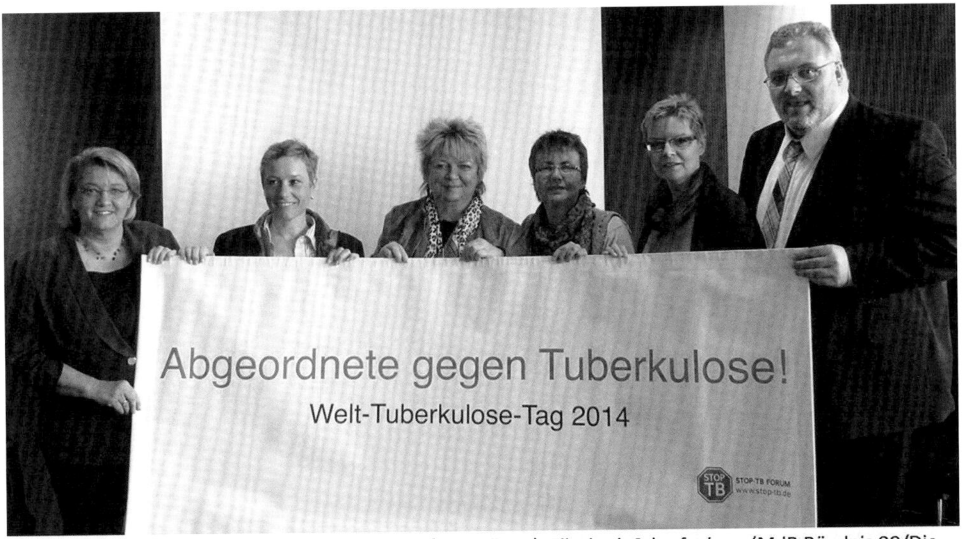
Abgeordnete gegen Tuberkulose!
Welt-Tuberkulose-Tag 2014
STOP TB
STOP-TB FORUM

V.l.n.r.: Kordula Schulz-Asche (MdB Bündnis 90/Die Grünen), Elisabeth Scharfenberg (MdB Bündnis 90/Die Grünen), Mechthild Rawert (MdB SPD), Kathrin Vogler (MdB Die Linke), Sabine Dittmar (MdB SPD), Erich Irlstorfer (MdB CDU/CSU)

Fig.1 German Parliamentarians at a breakfast which the Stop-TB Forum organized on the occasion of the World-TB-Day 2014

secures synergies and a broader view of problems related with TB but also strengthens the visibility of the advocacy-network.

The Stop-TB Forum works closely together with other German NGOs doing advocacy in health and HIV/Aids. It also works together with international actors that include and empower grassroot organizations from high TB-burden countries like the Stop TB Partnership and the TB Europe Coalition.

b) engages with parliamentarians and other political actors in Germany about TB

The Stop-TB Forum discusses with political actors about TB and organizes events, like parliamentarian breakfasts, which inform political decision makers about the global health threat of TB and the needs of the people affected by the disease.

c) informs the public in Germany about TB

The Stop-TB Forum provides information and organizes public events to inform the public about TB and to raise public awareness of the global health problem the disease poses.

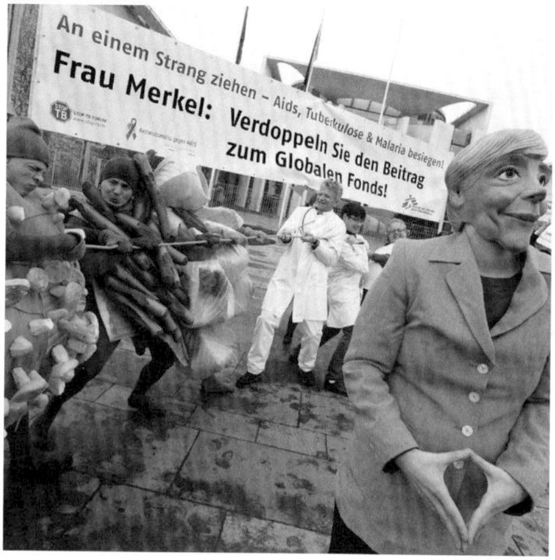

Fig.2 Public Stunt of the Stop-TB Forum together with Action against Aids and Doctors Without Borders, December 2013

d) conducts research and provides information.

The Stop-TB Forum also provides information about TB. Currently the network is conducting a study which will map the different actors working on the topic in Germany.

Author

Stop-TB Forum
c/o Ärzte ohne Grenzen e.V.
Am Köllnischen Park 1
10179 Berlin
Tel.: +49-30-700 130 192
Mobil: +49-176-988 13 131
www.stop-tb.de

The Akkon University for Human Sciences would like to thank all authors for their excellent contributions and for agreeing to invest much additional efforts to change a presentation into a written manuscript. In the long process of working on the current first issue of Akkon Schriftenreihe, the manuscripts underwent several updates and links to current developments in the fields of both tuberculosis control and global antibiotic resistance control. At the end, the first issue of the Akkon Schriftenreihe fulfills one of its tasks, namely contributing to current discussions in humanitarian aid, development aid and global health.

The Akkon University for Human Sciences would also like to thank for the generous financial support provided by Janssen Cilag GmbH and by Becton Dickinson Diagnostics.

akkon

hochschule für
humanwissenschaften